DOES GETTING OLD SCARE YOU ?

Introduction

I0414137

This Book was inspired by the little voice inside that directs our lives. Everyone has that little voice, some listen and take the suggestions, and some do not. I have found over the years that things work out better for me, if I follow the little voice suggestions. I have not always taken the suggestions, but this time I did. I was supposed to write a book and the title was given to me, Does Getting Old Scare You? Since I am old and hopefully getting older, I thought this should be fairly easy. I was wrong. I have written things before, I even wrote quite a bit to do my job, but my previous writings had a fairly focused theme. This was a little different. My focus was to keep the book short and informative. The short part was what gave me trouble. I brought up issues in the book that could take a life of their own and be spun off into a complete book by itself. Avoiding this pit fall was difficult. The little voice even selected the book cover. As I was searching for an image that might work I was led to an unexpected web-site www turnbacktogod.com which is the source of the photo.

DOES GETTING OLD SCARE YOU ?

This book was written and published for the sole purpose of sharing information and ideas. The hope is to spark the reader's interest to the point that they assess their life style as it pertains to their health and well-being.

In this book, you will see phrases repeated, that is because I feel these statements are important enough to warrant repeating it helps emphasize the issue.

DOES GETTING OLD SCARE YOU ?

About the Author/ Disclaimer

I, the author, E. J. Cain am not a health care professional but just an every day lady who has lived long and cared for family members and family pets. Some of the family members did not enjoy good health before they died, requiring in-home health care. This means you become an honorary "Nurse" /Vet by default.

You should not consider the material in this book to be the practice of medicine. However, a lot of the statements made in this book came from years of researching published medical literature and reports from prestigious Medical Schools, Clinics and hospitals.

 I have also received Publications and patient testimonials from Medical doctors who moved their practice in the Alternative direction many years ago. Needless to say, most of the information being shared was attained from life. I have also exchanged numerous conversations with people who use and support Alternative Medicine that I also support. In my life, I have lived in Europe for 8 years and traveled a lot. I have also traveled a lot inside the USA.

DOES GETTING OLD SCARE YOU ?

I am currently a Senior Citizen in good health.

I have done extensive research on Alternative and Holistic Medicine from around the world to see what folks do to maintain good health. I grew up in rural Western Colorado where doctors were few are far between, and grandma took care of the family ailments with natural home remedies. Some of grandma's other patients were farm animals and pets.

DOES GETTING OLD SCARE YOU ?

Table of Contents:

DOES GETTING OLD SCARE YOU ?

The title of the book, asks the question; does getting old scare you?   If you are over 50, your answer should be yes.   If it doesn't, scare you, it should at least give you a pause for thought about where you are in your life.

 I am writing this book to share information that I have learned over my many years. I have also done a lot of research and have drawn some conclusions on what works and what doesn't about staying healthy as we age.

 Old, how do we define it?   Old is one of those ambiguous words that mean something different to each person.   Maybe the question should be "are you afraid of becoming a Senior Citizen". However, that term is also a little ambiguous.   Society in the USA has an age range that they define as Senior Citizens. It often begins as early as 55 when some retail merchants offer Senior Citizens monetary discounts on their purchases. Senior Citizens carry this handle for a number of years until they reach their 100th birthday, at which point the label changes to Centenarian Citizen and there are not too many of those.

DOES GETTING OLD SCARE YOU ?

I have heard Senior adults comment that,
"growing old is not for sissies. " Since I have
observed many Seniors face some large health
obstacles and overcome them, I would agree
with that statement.

However, I personally did not consider myself
as a Senior until I was forced into the U.S.
Medicare system under the U.S. government
rules. I did, however, accept any Senior
discounts offered by retail merchants.

Growing old is often associated with dying.
Every person who is born ultimately knows that
at some point, they are going to die. However,
most people do not even think about dying until
they are older or their health starts to decline.
Fear of dying may scare some folks. However,
the fear of dying is different from the fear of
growing old. Growing old usually happens
gradually and each individual's body ages
differently. Growing old means living with "all"
the changes your body is going through on a
daily basis and it is more pleasant for some than
others.

DOES GETTING OLD SCARE YOU ?

So when do these little changes start?   Or really, how did we begin this "adventure" called human "life"?

In the beginning, God made man in his own image. He made them to reign over the other animal species of the earth.   God made a man "Adam" and a woman "Eve". God designed the human body to live forever.   Then a Snake talked Eve into eating the forbidden apple from the tree of life, and Eve convinced Adam the fruit was good.

 This is when "Sin," first" entered the picture and it angered God so much that he kicked Adam and Eve out of the Garden of Eden.

This is when our chronological bodies were changed forever. That is because "death" and a lot of other bad things came with "Sin".

Even though Adam was thrown out of the Garden, he did manage to live to the ripe old age of 930.   Bible scripture tells us God revised man's life span to 120 years. (Genesis: 6, 3).

DOES GETTING OLD SCARE YOU ?

 Then follow-up   Bible scripture (Psalms: 90, 10) states that 70 years is all we have, 80 if we are strong.   Since we have seen a number of people who have lived way beyond 80 years, all we really know for sure is that humans are not " immortal".

As human beings, we start our lives as an embryo inside our mother's uterus.
 During the next 9-months we develop into a baby before being born into the world. Everything our Mom is eating or exposed to while we are in the womb becomes a part of the body's building blocks of life and structure. Depending on the Mom, this can be good or bad. At birth the normal baby usually has all of the parts a body needs to exist, however, it takes the baby child about 20 years to fully develop mentally, physically and emotionally.

 Male and female humans are very different physically, emotionally and mentally and as such their road to maturity is a little different.

Their biological clocks are definitely on a different maturity trajectory. Females often mature before males.

DOES GETTING OLD SCARE YOU ?

Generally, females have all of their physical height by age 16, where males often continue to grow in height into their early 20s.

Girth, for both Male and Females, can be gained or lost at any age as girth is directly associated with the eating behavior and activity of the person, excluding any medical related issues.

A lot of kids become more age sensitive as they approach their teenage years.

It is in the teenage years that the Male and Female body identities really take form and show their differences.   It is at this time that the Males and Females undergo huge hormonal changes. This is really the beginning of hormonal changes that drive us through life. Hormonal changes affect the whole body, physically, mentally and emotionally. Physical changes are identified more quickly due to the physical appearance and emotions are often not quite as visible. Mental changes are not usually as visible to the onlooker.

DOES GETTING OLD SCARE YOU ?

Some of the identifying physical changes that occur are: Males and Females begin to grow hair under their arms on their legs and in their genital regions.
Males even grow hair on their buttocks! Most Males begin to grow facial hair and their voices change to a lower octave.   Hair is often grown between the eyebrows on Females and some even grow facial hair as well.

Sexuality is normally activated during these years. Society has put a name label on these changes, and they call it, "Puberty".

There have even been quite a few books written on the subject; "What's Happening To Me" was the book we bought for our boys when they were approaching Puberty.
These changes do not happen over night, and are often in a constant state of flux for about 3 to 5 years.   Timing is different for each individual. Heredity and nutrition play a role in the timing.   As you get older, you realize that "Puberty" is really the first pivotal point of your life.

I believe we go through four major pivot points in our life before you get to be a Centenarian.

DOES GETTING OLD SCARE YOU ?

With each pivotal point, your body goes through some type of major change either physically or mentally or both.

For most people, the birthday anxiety normally starts to decline by your 21st birthday.   By age 25, birthdays are not near as important as they once were. Unless your body is out of the normal range for whatever reason, by age 25 your wisdom teeth should be in and if you're a Male you should have reached your full height. Hopefully a little wisdom came with your wisdom teeth.

At this point your body has reached its prime and has physically peaked.

Medical schools and foundations have conducted quite a lot of research with published reports on how the body ages and every year more information is discovered.

Since our bodies are mortal, how we age has become a very popular subject. Popularity often breeds greed, so there are a lot of "snake oil" salesmen out there selling youthful products and the Internet has made it easier than ever to get the word out.

DOES GETTING OLD SCARE YOU ?

Society should tell you to enjoy your 20s, because after age 29 the subtle changes to your body each year become a little more pronounced.

You recognize the physical changes going on, but rarely notice your mental growth at this age.   Research has shown that your body even starts to lose some of the things it needs to stay vibrant.   Skin actually starts to decline in your mid-20s.   Skin even declines sooner if it has been exposed direct sunlight for long periods of time with out proper protection.

These are the years when you are deciding what you're going to do with your life, and obtain the additional education or training to accomplish your goals.

What your body may go through in your Senior years is not even on your radar, but it should be.

These are also the years that some people experiment with recreational drugs, consume alcohol in excess, and consume food that is not very healthy.   At this time, we often deny the body of the 8 hours of sleep needed for peak performance, and body restoration, which is done while we sleep.

DOES GETTING OLD SCARE YOU ?

There are some people that continue this 20s life style way into their 30s.   These years are full of "stress". Some folks recognize it and some don't, but either way your body has experienced "stress" which affects the body's overall health negatively.

Then by age 39 the body is going through another pivotal point in your life, and one more time, hormones are the culprits.   Even if you did not recognize the changes in your 20s, people can usually feel this round of hormone fluctuation.
This is why some people will only admit to being 39 for many years after they have gone past that birthday.

For most people, it is during their 40s that the hormones start raging once again.
Society also has a label for this round also and it is called "change of life " (Females) or mid-life crisis usually associated with the Males.

No matter what label you put on these changes, hormones are involved once again.   The hormones in our body regulate practically everything.

DOES GETTING OLD SCARE YOU ?

Not just your sex organs and your hair and skin…. but your heartbeat, your respiration, your bone growth and your sleep patterns. When your hormones are in balance, your body is too. However, when your hormones are out of whack, all kinds of bad things can happen to your body.   Therefore, to remain in good health, it is prudent to keep your hormones in harmony. This is often harder than it sounds.

Research labs tell us that our metabolism begins slowing down in our 30s. By the time we reach 40 a slow metabolism is in full bloom.

Your body gaining weight for no apparent reason without doing anything differently is one of the signs.   We have hot flashes and night sweats. Our temperament often changes as well, and it is not just Females that experience these things.   Even though it is often identified with the Females more.

These years are often very busy ones. Your kids are now teenagers or they are headed off to College with a need for extra money.   A few in today's society have even waited to start a family until their early 40s.

DOES GETTING OLD SCARE YOU ?

The Family budget is often in conflict with saving money for retirement and paying for day-to-day necessities. The bottom line is you have a lot going on.

By your mid 40s you are either a success in your chosen career, or you still may be looking for your niche in life, and buying lottery tickets as a means of obtaining your fortune. Your hair may be turning gray or even thinning, or you may have even lost some or all of it. Either way, these are the kind of things that cause "Stress".

Or maybe you have discovered that you are at peace with yourself just the way you are, which is less stressful. In your 40s is when you notice a loss of physical energy and stamina.

Doctors are quick to check our hearts, focus on cholesterol levels, weight and blood pressure and prescribe medications for these symptoms if they are out of the normal range.

However, I think stress is at the root of a lot of the things we have going on and is under rated by our medical society.

DOES GETTING OLD SCARE YOU ?

It is very hard on a body's over all health and can cause a variety of illnesses.

Stress can come at any age for a number of reasons, but it seems to pick up speed in the 40s because this is when we realize we are not going to get younger.

Society has compartmented us by age and has even associated a list of things that should have been accomplished by a certain age.

Some folks even get 'stressed,' if they feel they are out of their compartmented zone.

I do not believe the medical profession adequately informs our middle age people about the dangers that "stress" poses to their health. In the past 20 years "Stress" has been added to the list of various names, e.g. trouble sleeping, tension head aches, digestive problems to name a few.

Most people are exposed to some kind of stress when they are young, however, for most people the body seems to deal with it better when we are young.

DOES GETTING OLD SCARE YOU ?

Through it all, somehow you have made it to age 50 and you are slowing down a little more. You still feel young, but you notice you cannot get as much done during the day, as you once did. Sometimes just mowing the grass causes you to search for one of the liniments you've seen advertised.

With that 50th birthday, comes a medical protocol that suggests people start getting in-depth annual physicals. This is also when doctors want to do EKG for the heart and multiple blood tests. This is also when the doctor insists on a colonoscopy test. These tests will inform us how our body is doing.

These tests are for the healthy person. If you have a family history of medical issues, the tests begin sooner.

If you are still trying to live the same life style that you did in your 30s, your body will be protesting. This is the time folks get strokes, arthritis, heart attacks and a menagerie of other ailments.

DOES GETTING OLD SCARE YOU ?

As you get older your body's arteries begin to stiffen and pick up a little plaque. Your current or past life styles can accelerate the aging process or even make it worse.

After age 50 most people find it harder to stay in good physical shape. Our body is inter-connected, so any change to one area can have a domino effect on the whole body.

There is a larger age range for the hormone shift that takes place in our 50s than there was for the Puberty change.
Heredity may be a small influence, but for most people, 50 years of life style is the dominant factor in this change. However, each individual is different.

It is often in the 50s that the Female body stops being able to produce the fertile eggs required to produce offspring, however, there are always a few exceptions. By contrast the Male body can still reproduce offspring for many years.

Because of these differences, a lot of men will not even want to admit they are going through any kind of life change or crisis.   These years represent another pivotal point in ones life.

DOES GETTING OLD SCARE YOU ?

If we looked deeper into the medical Research, we find that a lot of things that make up our body, like cells, proteins and enzymes are changing or declining with age.
The 50s is also the time, when any of the ailments the body might have, mental or physical become more active and visible.

It is in the late 40s and 50s that Males and Females even begin to think about their health. Most people's thinking is controlled by mob psychology. The average person has been trained to think falsely that as the years go by you are supposed to get old. The body is supposed to decline and deteriorate; to include the mind. The spirit seems not to be so defined. Age brings on troubles so they have been told and that is what they believe.
This type of thinking is why folks have been in search of the "fountain of youth" for centuries, without success.

Over the years there has been a lot of money made by those who advertise and sell their version of the "fountain of youth".

DOES GETTING OLD SCARE YOU ?

Television, magazine and Internet commercials are on display continually, but do not believe everything you hear and see.

The body is not immortal and "Dorian Gray" was just a fictional character in a book.

By your mid 50s you are eligible for "Senior" discounts at some retail merchants, "yea"!

By this age you are either planning your retirement, or you have figured out you will have to work until you die.

If you have to continue working, you may find it harder to get a good job.   Remember that "mob psychology"? Well a lot of employers share that attitude and they want younger people. With each birthday, it gets even harder.

This is the time when depression can set in if you are not careful.

But there is hope, some employers have had a bad experience with the younger generation's work ethic and actually want healthy older workers.

DOES GETTING OLD SCARE YOU ?

Some of you out there may even have had your children or grand children move back in with you. This can bring on a whole new set of issues for your life, some good and some bad. If your life situation becomes less than desirable, it can bring on a lot of negative "stress " that impacts your health.

If you have survived the 50s, you have now reached 60. You have been fairly healthy most of your life, but now you find that some of the foods you like really don't agree with you anymore.

You also find that what you used to like to drink, doesn't really agree with you either. Some of you may go to the Internet, some may even go to "WEBMD" and some may talk to a friend, some may even go off to the doctor to ask, "What is going on with your health." No matter where you go to for an answer; the end result is going to be the same.
Every answer is going to point you to change your life style in some form. If your search takes you to a doctor, they may even give you some pharmaceutical pills or recommend some supplements /vitamins.

DOES GETTING OLD SCARE YOU ?

 The doctor may also recommend a list of things to eat and drink, or a protocol to follow.

This may work for those of you who can follow what the doctor suggest, however, there are lot of people who have been doing things their way for so long, that they will not change. Each time they see their doctor, they say that they are trying to follow the rules, even though they know it is a lie.

These are the same folks that end up on a doctor merry-go-round and never really feel well, no matter what day it is.   Giving your doctor polite suggestions to help with diagnosis and knowing something about an illness can save you time and money and give you a greater chance for a quick recovery.

Society calls these years the "Golden Years". However, the truth is they are only golden if you have good health and a sufficient amount of money to do the things you want to do.
When you reach 65 you are officially considered "old". You are forced onto the government directed health care system called Medicare for your health care.

DOES GETTING OLD SCARE YOU ?

Maybe you have had a good medical plan during your working years, but now you are forced into Medicare.   The bad news is, not all doctors accept Medicare. Medicare covers very few of the procedures and therapies you need to stay healthy, as you get older.

They will cover chiropractor but only if you have had an injury, it does not cover periodic maintenance.   If you go to the chiropractor for an alignment to stay aligned and healthy, they won't pay.

Medicare does not cover massage therapy, acupuncture or any energy healing therapies, that might keep you healthy; but they will cover surgery and expensive medications. If a doctor recommends Therapeutic Massage for a specific ailment, they may cover a little of that cost. Medicare will pay for some vitamins, if the doctor prescribes them for your health.

Medicare pays very little for preventative treatments, except for some immunization shots.

DOES GETTING OLD SCARE YOU ?

Let me reiterate, Medicare will not pay for prevention of disease or declining health, but they will pay for surgery and pharmaceutical medications after you get the disease or body ailment.

Something is definitely wrong with that logic. Even when Medicare does pay, it is only a portion of the costs., usually about 80%.   This means you have to obtain additional medical insurance out of your pocket in addition to the monthly premium you pay for Medicare, or pay the cash difference.

Sometimes, even when you have additional insurance, you still may have to pay cash out of pocket.

The rules for Medicare are many and change every year so you must keep up to date.

Some surgeries and procedures that might be recommended by the Medical Community when you are younger, are not recommended, as you get older. Hence, these procedures are not covered or paid by Medicare.

DOES GETTING OLD SCARE YOU ?

The thing about growing old is that it comes on gradually and you do not even realize it.
 Which is probably where the old saying "Young at Heart, other parts slightly older" comes from.

Oh, occasionally when you really look into a mirror and question to whom does that face belong, that is looking back at you. However, the mind often plays tricks on us; and the face you see is that of a point in time when you were happy or comfortable with the way you look. This could explain why we look at recently taken photos and say, "is that really me"? I guess this might be where the saying of, " in the mind's eye" comes from.

There is another saying out there from a German philosopher, Friedrich Nietzsche; "That which does not kill us, ...Makes us stronger".

When our body is exposed to small amounts of things that would normally hurt or kill us, whether it is chemical, emotional or physical it can actually make us stronger. This principle is kind of the basis for allergy shots.

DOES GETTING OLD SCARE YOU ?

In general Seniors only truly feel old if their health, physically or mentally, has declined. Some of them even remember doing cartwheels and all sorts of things they did in their youth, but at same time their reality turns on and says I cannot do that today. It is funny how those things come and go. I guess you could say the body ages, but in your heart you are forever young.

The medical arena is not the only place where Seniors are treated differently. Remember that "mob psychology" attitude I mentioned earlier, that says Seniors decline mentally and physically with age. Well that attitude is now on full display.

The bottom line is that turning 65 puts a target on you, for those who try to take advantage of the weak, mentally challenged and the elderly. The Internet has made it harder for those who have been placed on Medicare, or if you have signed up for Social Security to keep their age a secret, because they are now in a Federal Government database. For those of you that fall in these categories, you know what I mean.

DOES GETTING OLD SCARE YOU ?

You remember getting all of the un-solicited mail from insurance companies wanting you to buy their Insurance plan in lieu of government Medicare. These companies have made a deal with Medicare to provide you medical services.

If you sign up for one of these plans, that insurance company will get X amount of dollars each month from the government Medicare office. That insurance company will then make the decisions on what and how much they will pay for your medical costs. Some of these companies restrict your coverage to specified clinics and doctors. So when you are making your decisions be sure you investigate all your options before selecting your Medicare provider. Some folks just stay with the government Medicare, which is the choice I made. I found this one to be more flexible, and less rules.

You also get inundated with insurance companies wanting to sell you a Supplemental insurance plan to cover the costs that Medicare does not pay. Then of course there are a sundry of other companies looking for Senior customers to buy, walkers, scooters, walking canes and other such items.

DOES GETTING OLD SCARE YOU ?

Scam artists also prey on Seniors.   Then there are the Donation seekers who approach Seniors frequently.

Thugs attack Seniors on the street, or even go to their homes because the thinking is that older people are more vulnerable.

The television watching generations seem to have been Brainwashed into believing the pharmaceutical companies have a "Magic Pill" for anything that ails you.   There are some Seniors on this pharmaceutical merry-go-around.

While they are on this recipe for optimum health, there are some Seniors that feel the medical community is actually using them to test the new pharmaceutical medications.

These are the same people that have either forgotten or they were never taught that God made our bodies as his temple for us to take care of properly.   So if we treat our body with respect and take care of properly, it is designed to heal and repair itself.

DOES GETTING OLD SCARE YOU ?

Undergoing Cranial Sacral Therapy really shows you how the body wants to respond with very little encouragement.
This is a Therapy that can be started on babies and done through out your life.

I am a firm believer in this Therapy for health, because the body does want to heal itself.

Continuing on with the financial exploitation of Seniors:

If you have had a health issue that required you to go to a hospital for even a short stay, and it is a "non profit" hospital you may get contacted by that organization for a donation or even suggest you put them in your will.

Some Lending institutions even make their financial information so complex that it can mislead anyone, especially Seniors.

The old jokes you have heard over the years about old folks being blind, senile, and without memory, are not jokes when "they " are now referring to you without knowing you.

DOES GETTING OLD SCARE YOU ?

One more time, they are making assumptions based on the societal "mob psychology" compartmental averages once again.

If you are this age, you must have these things wrong with you, which may or may not be true. This is could be why, as a Senior person, you become concerned when folks ask you questions like, are you sure you are up to driving your car that far? Or do you need someone to go to the doctor with you to interpret what the doctor is telling you.

Or do you need help with operating, gadget A, B, or C. They might even ask if you need help making purchase decisions.

Even if you think you are doing fine, these types of questions, make you stop and think; "what do these younger people think is going on with me"?

You ask yourself if you might have done something to lead them to believe you need help, or if they are just counting your birthdays. You might even doubt yourself, or some may even feel insecure.

DOES GETTING OLD SCARE YOU ?

Most of you never had these feelings when you were younger.   If you do not have a close relationship with your "God", it can be scary.

Adults in their 20s and 30s usually have good health, high energy and not so much wisdom.

After age 60 your energy has probably slowed down and your health may be declining, but your wisdom is better than that of a 20 year old.

 However, wisdom is often accompanied with wrinkles and gray hair; so you will most likely face resistance trying to convince younger folks of that increased wisdom phenomenon.

As you reminisce your life experiences, you find yourself reminding younger folks, that a person does not always get "do-overs", for bad life style health decisions that are made in your youth.

However by the time Senior age approaches; you have figured out that you cannot change the past; you just have to live with the result of any bad life style choices, and deal with the way you are at this point.

DOES GETTING OLD SCARE YOU ?

As a young child, you usually think that Seniors should be treated with dignity and honored for their wisdom.

This was true when I was young, but I do not believe that this is still true today in America. I was trying to remember when Senior respect started to decline.

This has been another one of those gradual things and it appears to coincide with taking God out of our lives and Country.
Remember one of God's Commandment's is to honor our mother and father.

The electronic devices we engage with daily in lieu communicating with family and friends has added to the disconnect we have in the true fellowship and bonding with one another. The Bible tells us to honor our elders, so religious families tend to do better in this regard than the non-religious folks do.

Several Countries around the world still honor the elderly in their society. Some Countries still believe it is the oldest Son's responsibility to take care of the parents in their Senior years, usually in his family home.

DOES GETTING OLD SCARE YOU ?

When people from all over the world first migrated to America they brought those types of customs with them.

Some Americans still hold to those values for Seniors.   However, there are a large number of folks who feel they have zero responsibility for the elderly.   Maybe these are the folks that were dropped off at daycare at a very early age with their formative years being influenced by "whoever" was at the daycare, in lieu of Grandma or a family member.   There are even those in America, that feel Seniors should not live with their children in their declining years.

This thought process has been so ingrained into our Society that Seniors are encouraged by Retirement Planners to include saving dollars for a "nursing or assisted living facility" should one be needed.

In America we even have a Medicaid system, paid for by taxpayers, to put Seniors in "nursing homes" for those who cannot afford it.   This program does very little investigation to see if the family of the senior could afford to pay for the nursing home, they just bill it to the taxpayer.

DOES GETTING OLD SCARE YOU ?

There are families that have even had legal documents implemented on the Senior assets to insure the Senior would qualify for taxpayer assisted living. Something just sounds morally wrong with this concept.

 But the net result is that Seniors can be placed in nursing homes for someone other than family members to provide for their care.

By contrast, there are some middle age families, who work outside the home for a living, that have to drop off the kids at daycare and then take their Senior family member to a facility that takes care of Seniors who can not stay by themselves during the day. All of this effort just to get to work.
There are even some that also have to drop a pet off for daily care. These types of families are honorable and few and far between.

If you are the 60 to 70 year old being taken to day care every day like a child, it is a very emotional experience. At some level you recognize that it is putting a burden on the whole family.

DOES GETTING OLD SCARE YOU ?

You are proud and thankful that your family loves you this much. Some folks can adapt and accept what is happening every day in their life, others cannot.

If you have not been close with "God"/ "higher power" in your life, this would be good time to find him and pray for strength to deal with life. Chances are, you are going to be stuck in this mode until you die.
The bottom line is that growing old gets a little scary after age 60. It is scarier if you have bad health.   Chances are good that you have already buried your parents.

You can plan for the Senior years, and the road to get there.   The one thing that is known is that the road will lead to death at some point, you just won't know when.

The unknown is that you never know what kind of turns are going to be in your road or at what point in your life they will come.

Here are some possible turns your road could take:

DOES GETTING OLD SCARE YOU ?

 If you have been married for several years and your spouse dies, life can get real emotional and stressful.

 Stress is a double edge sword. It can cause a health issue, or the health issue can cause Stress.   Therefore, the earlier in life you learn to manage stress the better off you are. Loss of a spouse could also mean a loss of monetary support.

Or one spouse can even come down with an illness requiring the other spouse to take care of them. These are   scenarios that plague the elderly more than the young.

We live in a mobile society, and Seniors sometimes lose their mobility. Just getting around the house can be challenging. Loss of the ability to drive can devastate some Seniors, particularly if you live in the country. The older you get the chances are greater for loosing friends and even children to death.   You begin to feel very isolated.

You love the younger folks, but you do not feel the common bond with them that you do with people close to your age, I am not sure why, but my association with other Seniors seem to support this belief.

DOES GETTING OLD SCARE YOU ?

This is why you see many Seniors move into Senior Retirement Communities.

Florida is a state that has a lot of Senior Living Communities. Senior Living Communities are popping up in many states now as the "baby boomers" are retiring.

If you really do not want to move into a Senior Living Community, or your circumstances will not permit it, there are other things you can do to provide you similar experiences.

 Most communities have Senior Centers. Senior Centers usually act as the conduit for group activities that often provide entertainment and enrichment for Seniors.   It can also be the place where Seniors gather to share their life experiences, share pictures of the grandkids or just talk about life in general.

The cost to operate these centers is usually paid by the city, so any fees to do activities are usually very minimal and varies from Center to Center. Most towns and cities have clubs and organizations that might appeal to you as well; and of course most towns have churches to join.

DOES GETTING OLD SCARE YOU ?

The bottom line is that you do not have to be by yourself all the time, even if you have limited resources.

People really prefer to reminiscence with people who share the same nostalgia and interests.

Since it is inescapable that if you live, you are going to get older. It would be nice to know a few things that could make the aging process a more pleasant experience.

First of all, when you have reached the age when you recognize that there is a direct correlation between how you feel and how you have treated your body, that is the time for you to take charge of your body on a daily basis.

We start with the basics, whatever we consume orally, or whatever your skin is exposed to, or whatever you inhale, effects your body in some way; whether you recognize it at the time or not.

DOES GETTING OLD SCARE YOU ?

We, here in the United States, had created government agencies to protect us, or so we thought. In 1848 the Food And Drug Administration, (FDA) was established. In 1862 the Department of Agriculture was created to watch over our food source.

Then in 1906 our government created the Pure Food and Drug Act to monitor our food and drug source. With all of these Federal groups watching out for us, we assume that the food and drugs we are purchasing are safe for consumption. In a perfect world this would be true, however, a perfect world does not exist. The bottom line is one has to be vigilant about one's health and do your own research.

While we are doing our research on what is best to put in our body we often run into challenges caused by our government.

The USA is a capitalistic country, which is good, but with capitalism also comes greed. Greed gives rise to "wheeler-dealer" type folks who know the definition of urgency.

DOES GETTING OLD SCARE YOU ?

Their urgency is tied to their profits. Wheeler-dealers can be very innovative and might even try to bribe or manipulate government officials into endorsing their product or idea for public consumption.

Problems can arise from having these large bureaucracies running your food and drug supplies.

They can create regulatory burdens and install processes that hinder the ability for suppliers to obtain the best food and drugs in a timely manner for the citizens. Urgency is not a word in a bureaucrat's dictionary.

When it comes to food, simple and natural is best. If you cannot pronounce what is on the food label and have zero idea of what it is, chances are, it won't help your body.

However, the computer has made it a lot easier to look the ingredients up so you can make your own decisions. There is new evidence that comes out frequently on what our bodies really need to operate well.

DOES GETTING OLD SCARE YOU ?

So it is prudent that you pay attention to the news that is coming out. Some of the things they put out in the 1960s, 1970s and 1980s have been debunked, particularly when it comes to fat and sugar in our diets.

A majority of the Senior patients visiting the doctor are using Medicare or some other type of insurance. Medical Insurance Companies are very regulated, either by the government or by their own internal policies and procedures. These regulations often hamper the doctor's ability to run the type of tests needed to determine the "root cause" of your ailment. Exceptions are sometimes made, if your doctor is unable to manage your symptoms via pharmaceuticals.

Pharmaceuticals may not be the solution to cure your ailment; as a lot of pharmaceuticals are designed more to manage your symptoms, not provide a cure, e.g. blood pressure pills.

DOES GETTING OLD SCARE YOU ?

It is left up to you and your doctor to learn what kind of nutrition and exercise that your body needs for optimum health. These findings can be the solution for many of your health disorders.

The doctor's schedule is limited and they often see several patients per day.

This type of environment does not allow the doctor time for in-depth research for each patient. This is when you have to recognize that you are the one that has to take charge of getting your body well.

If you don' t take the time or interest; then your health could be doomed. After all, you live in your body every day, and most of us only see the doctor occasionally. Since it is your body, you are more aware of what is going on with it; than your doctor does. You also have a greater interest in finding out what your body needs for optimum health.

If you are unable to do your own research, you can probably find someone who can help you. Word of mouth from friends and family and the computer are very good sources for research.

DOES GETTING OLD SCARE YOU ?

Libraries are also very helpful in finding medical publications from Medical Schools, Clinics and Universities.

Pharmaceuticals are only a band-aid for immediate and temporary relief. Non-pharmaceutical creams and substances can also provide the same temporary relief.

However, they do not get to the "root cause" of what created your problem. Until you find the "root cause" of the problem and deal with that issue, it will not permanently go away. If the "root cause" cannot be found, or dealt with, for whatever reason, then you are stuck with temporary fixes.

There are some people who would rather do temporary fixes than put out the effort and money to get to the root cause of their ailment.

For some people it's the money and for others it is just plain laziness. No matter which of the two reasons it is, it provides the Pharmaceutical Industry with an opportunity to sell you "something" to give you temporary relief for your ailment.

DOES GETTING OLD SCARE YOU ?

The pharmaceutical industry has been advertising on television for several years now. They have told people they need this pill or that pill for nearly everything your body might wakeup with that hurt or that does not work properly.

There are even folks out there that believe that their doctor has a "Magic Pill" for everything.

It is unbelievable that people can watch an ad for a drug, hear the "whole" ad with what the drug can do for you; then hear the "long" list of potential drug side effects that are often quite dastardly, and miss the side effects altogether. Which only re-enforces the old saying, "that people only hear what they want to hear."

These same people will go to their doctor and demand these drugs; and the doctors who are short on time, will often prescribe the pills requested. It is truly amazing. People who believe these ads and take the pills repeatedly are often the same people with poor health and degraded memory.

DOES GETTING OLD SCARE YOU ?

Seniors can also get caught in a loop if they have an accident or surgery   to repair disorders that affect their mobility.

 After the surgery the doctor will normally require the patient to go to a rehab facility for a period of time to recover and get therapy. These facilities are often co-located with a long-term care facility. The rehab centers are not cheap.

These facilities have a "protocol" in place to rehab the patients. These "protocols" often include a substantial amount of Pharmaceutical drugs.   Their goal is to keep the patient comfortable and pain free.

The body has just been cut on, so there is pain, and now the Physical Therapist wants them to exercise that limb that has just been repaired by a Surgeon.   You have guessed it. That "hurts", so the rehab center offsets the pain with " Narcotic pain killer " that turns the pain off in the brain.

DOES GETTING OLD SCARE YOU ?

It does not just effect the brain, it effects the whole body and shuts down organs that you need to operate properly e.g. kidneys and bowels.

There are several "Opioid (Narcotics)" on the market today. You may recognize them by their name; Codeine, Morphine, Hydrocodone, and Oxycodone are a few. Doctors have found that when some folks used these drugs for an injury/disorder, they get addicted to them.

The news outlets sometimes cover these drug-addicted reports when a celebrity is involved, like Elvis Presley or Michael Jackson.
These pills are expensive, so the Pharmaceutical Industry will not be discouraging the use of their pills any time soon.

The Internet is covered with stories of the overuse of "Opioids" becoming an Epidemic in the USA.   Opioids are a very close cousin to the illegal drugs like "Heroin".

DOES GETTING OLD SCARE YOU ?

So Seniors it is up to you one more time to take charge of your health care.

 When you are in these rehab centers be vigilant of the medications you are receiving. If you are in a facility that is co-located with a long-term care, take a hard look at people in long-term care and see if you really want to be there. Or do you just want the Therapy and to go home recovered?   If you do a little research on the folks that are in long-term care, you will find it is people that never learned how to deal with or take charge of their physical, mental or emotional stress when they were young. A lot of these folks are in the "woe is me crowd", requesting the doctor give them a "Magic Pill".

I think a visit to these long-term care homes, would provide teenagers a good visual on what happens to you when you do not "Take Charge" of your body and health at an early age.

DOES GETTING OLD SCARE YOU ?

What do I mean when I say "Take Charge," that means you consider everything your body is exposed to; liquid intake to include water, any nutrients you eat or take in pill or powder form.

You watch for everything your skin touches, to include spiders and mosquitos. It includes the oils, creams and lotions you put on your skin and the water you use to bathe or shower.

And what do these "hand sanitizers" really have in them? I personally avoid these and use Essential Three Thieves Oil instead. At least I can spell and say what is in them, plus they have a history of success for killing germs for over 500 years. If you believe in the Bible, there are several oils identified for health issues in it. The oils people remember most are Frankincense and Myrrh, because of their association with Christmas, as these were the oils the Three Wisemen presented as gifts to the baby Jesus.

Reminder!!

Pharmaceuticals should be used for a short time to correct an acute problem, not a life long fix. Every Pharmaceutical drug has some type of side affect.

DOES GETTING OLD SCARE YOU ?

Those side affects can accumulate in your body over the years, and become a health issue itself.

Other things that you are exposed to over the years are also accumulative to the body, e.g. too much bright sun, bee stings, spider bites etc can also cause health issues. It is amazing how just a little tick bite can make you so sick. Tick bites are definitely accumulative to the body. At what age does the body say, "I have had all of that substance I can deal with".

The age depends on how many times the body has been exposed to a substance. It also depends on how well you detoxify your body. Old Timers used to have a ritual to detox every spring, with a concoction that Grandma prepared.

In general, these rituals have really gone by the wayside.

However, people who attempt to keep their body running good, normally have some type of detox ritual that they do periodically, or as they feel the body needs it.

DOES GETTING OLD SCARE YOU ?

<u>In Summary...</u>

Getting old is scary!!

It is less scary if you make good decisions, physically, mentally and emotionally when you are younger and have good health in your Senior years.

A person needs to learn early in life, that they need to take charge of their health. You are the only one that can do this.

If you believe in "God" or a higher power, relying on them for support is very reassuring and helpful. Religious people seem to grow old more gracefully. Maybe they believed the Bible, when it says God made your body as a temple and you are to respect and take care of that temple.

Remember if you go into a hospital or any facility treating the sick and dying, that all of the people there are not strong believers in God.

DOES GETTING OLD SCARE YOU ?

The devil sends "evil spirits" to these places to get your soul while you are in a vulnerable state. I have always felt better in these facilities when there is a Chapel in the building. I also like to see the Clergy walking the halls visiting folks.

True Religious people are not usually afraid to die, because they believe at death they will be going to live with Jesus in a perfect place.

However, if their health is bad, getting older is a little scary for them also.

I have read that: "The Best Classroom in the world, is at the feet of an elderly person.

Good Health is the Key to have good life adventures.

www.ingramcontent.com/pod-product-compliance
Lightning Source LLC
Chambersburg PA
CBHW050521290526
45786CB00007B/2640